I0782711

Knowing the Terrain

Communication is Sexier Than You Think

Before embarking on any adventure, talk to your partner. Ask what they like, what they'd rather avoid, and if they have any fantasies in mind. If you're unsure how to start, say something like, *"Do you have a special playlist for these moments... or are we improvising?"*

Confidence: Your Best Accessory

Nothing ignites passion more than someone who knows their worth. Walk into the bedroom like you're on a runway, but remember: there's a fine line between confidence and acting like a bad movie character.

Hygiene: The Real Prologue

A shower, fresh breath, and some personal care are essential. Romance dies when your partner wonders if that mysterious smell is coming from you or the couch.

Desire Has Its Own Timing

Don't get frustrated if your partner needs more or less time than you. Patience is key. Like a good chess game, the best move is to wait for the perfect moment.

The Art of Foreplay

Foreplay Starts Outside the Bedroom

Surprise your partner with a spicy text during the day or a stolen kiss in the kitchen. Great foreplay can begin hours before the main event, like a trailer that leaves you eager for the full movie.

Discover New Routes to Pleasure

Do you always aim for the obvious? Explore other erogenous zones. The back of the neck, wrists, even behind the knees... because the real adventure is in discovery.

Dirty Talk Has Its Science

Saying something provocative can be exciting, but do it tactfully. If you go for something out of a cheap novel, make sure your partner doesn't laugh at the wrong moment.

Anticipation Is Your Ally

Take your time; let the desire grow. Think of it as slow cooking: an exquisite dish takes time to prepare, but the wait is worth it.

The Main Event

Rhythm: Find the Right Melody

Going too fast can ruin everything, and too slow might make it seem like you're stuck thinking about the grocery list. Listen to the language of their sighs and adjust your rhythm as if you're performing a private concert.

Positions Aren't Just for the Kama Sutra

Experimenting is great, but remember you're not in an extreme yoga class. Find what works for both of you, and don't be afraid to laugh if something doesn't go as planned.

Hands Have a Lot to Say

Don't stick to basic movements. Explore, caress, and play, but avoid looking like a cat scratching new furniture.

Timing Is Everything

Finding the perfect moment to move or change things can make all the difference. Moving too early can lead to an uncoordinated choreography.

Eye Contact Is Powerful

An intense gaze at the right moment can be more erotic than any word. Just make sure you don't look like a mannequin staring into the distance.

Express Yourself Freely

Moans, sighs, or laughter: it's all allowed as long as it's genuine. Showing enjoyment is just as sexy as feeling it.

After the Act

Don't Disappear Like a Ninja

Sex doesn't end when it's over. A hug, light conversation, or even a *"Fancy some pizza?"* can prolong intimacy.

Be Generous with Compliments

After a great moment, don't be stingy with words. A *"That was amazing, how do you do it?"* always brings a smile.

Extras That Always Help

Be Spontaneous, But Not Intrusive

Suggesting something new can be exciting, but ensure you're on the same page. *"Let's try this"* works better than, *"Surprise! I brought a pirate costume!"*

Humor Saves Any Awkward Moment

If something goes wrong, laugh and move on. A good laugh is the best emotional lubricant.

Learn New Things
Reading, exploring, or simply asking your partner can open doors you didn't even know existed. Remember: sex is a journey, not a race.

The Key Moment

Strategic Pauses Are Essential

Stopping for a few seconds at the right moment can be more exciting than any continuous motion. Imagine you're a DJ pausing the best beat just before the climax—let the tension do its magic before continuing.

Be a Bold Explorer

Don't be afraid to suggest something new or let your partner take the lead and teach you what they enjoy. Think of it like being Indiana Jones—only instead of a lost temple, you're discovering the map to pleasure.

Don't Obsess Over the Finale

The climax is important, but it's not everything. Enjoy the journey, play with the texture of the moment, and remember: a good lover knows the journey is as pleasurable as the destination.

Incorporate All the Senses

It's not just about touch. Use sight, sound, taste, and smell. A whisper in the ear, a kiss that leaves a trail, or even a special perfume can add layers of intensity. And no, that bargain deodorant doesn't count as "special perfume."

Emotional Connection and the Aftermath

Affection Is the Dessert of Sex

A hug, a kiss, or simply lying together and staring at the ceiling can be just as satisfying as the act itself. Sometimes, a simple *"Want a glass of water?"* is more romantic than a poem.

Don't Be Afraid to Ask Questions

"Did you enjoy that?" or *"Anything you'd like to try next time?"* These questions not only show interest but also build trust and demonstrate that you're committed to improving. Plus, they can lead to interesting conversations—or even

more action.

Keep the Spark Alive Afterward

A flirty message the next day, an unexpected touch at a random moment, or even a simple *"I was thinking about last night"* can keep memories fresh.

Level Up with Extras

Be a Sexy Storyteller

Talking during sex doesn't always have to be dirty—it can be fun and sensual. Tell a little story or describe what you'd like to do next. Just make sure you don't sound like you're narrating an audiobook.

Stay Mentally Flexible

Maybe your partner wants to try something you've never considered. Keep an open mind and remember: a lover who adapts is unforgettable. Just ensure both of you are comfortable with the idea.

Mind the Atmosphere

Dim lights, soft music, or even a change of setting can transform the experience. But be careful with adventures in the kitchen—wooden chairs aren't always as romantic as they seem.

Don't Overlook the Small Gestures

Sometimes, a simple move like brushing their hair away from their face, wrapping them in a blanket afterward, or whispering their name can mean more than any elaborate technique.

Extras That Always Help

Be Spontaneous, but Not Intrusive

Suggesting something new can be exciting, but make sure you're on the same wavelength. *"Let's try this"* works better than, *"Surprise! I brought a pirate costume!"*

Humor Saves Any Awkward Moment

If something goes wrong, laugh it off and move forward. A good laugh is the best emotional lubricant.

Learn New Things
Reading, exploring, or simply asking your partner can open doors you didn't even know existed. Remember: sex is a journey, not a race.

The Key Moment

Strategic Pauses Are Essential

Stopping for a few seconds at the right moment can be more exciting than continuous motion. Think of yourself as a DJ pausing the best track just before the beat drops—let the anticipation work its magic before continuing.

Be a Bold Explorer

Don't be afraid to suggest something new or let your partner take the lead and show you what they enjoy. Think of it as being Indiana Jones, except instead of a lost temple, you're discovering the map to pleasure.

Don't Obsess Over the Finish Line

The climax is important, but it's not everything. Enjoy the journey, play with the texture of the moment, and remember: a great lover knows the journey is as pleasurable as the destination.

Engage All the Senses

It's not just about touch. Use sight, sound, taste, and smell. A whisper in the ear, a kiss that leaves a trail, or even a special scent can add layers of intensity. And no, that cheap deodorant doesn't count as a "special scent."

The Art of Rhythm and Timing

Subtle Rhythm Changes
Like a great song, alternating between soft and passionate moments keeps things interesting. Just don't switch so abruptly that it feels like you dropped the remote.

Trust Your Intuition
Pay attention to your partner's reactions: their breathing, movements, even their smile. You don't need an app to know if you're on the right track.

Endurance Isn't Everything

It's not a competition to see who lasts longer; it's about making every second count. Feel free to take a break, recharge, and return to the "battlefield" with a smile.

Spontaneity and Respect

Be Curious, But Respectful
Ask about fantasies or desires that your partner might not have shared before. Something as simple as, *"What would you like to try someday?"* can open doors to new experiences. But be cautious: if they mention skydiving,

make sure they're
speaking figuratively! ?

Use Your Voice as an Erotic Tool

A low, calm voice can be incredibly sensual. You don't need to be a nighttime radio host, but learn to whisper something sexy like you're sharing a secret only they should know. Just avoid sounding like you're narrating a nature documentary!

Know Your Limits and Theirs

A good lover knows not only what they can do but also when to stop. Trust is built when both partners feel safe to explore. Remember, even superheroes have their limits—no one wants to see you crash like a movie villain!

The Art of the "After" Doesn't End When You Get Up

If the moment was special, make it memorable all day long. A flirty message or a simple *"I can't stop thinking about you"* can be the bridge between a great encounter and the next one. Just don't send it

during their Zoom
meeting!

The Master Touch

Create Personal Rituals

A unique gesture that only you two share, like a kiss in a certain spot or a phrase before starting, can become a signal that ignites the flame instantly. Think of it as your own secret handshake—only sexier!

Add a Bit of Humor

Don't take yourself too seriously. A funny comment at the right moment can ease tension and make the experience feel more natural. But beware: telling jokes during the climax might throw off the rhythm!

Learn to Be Generous

Being a good lover isn't just about your own pleasure. Take time to discover what makes your partner happy and enjoy watching them experience it. Giving can be more satisfying than receiving—plus, it's harder to run out of things to give!

Feel Proud of the Moment

After a great session, don't be afraid to celebrate your success together. Just don't get too excited and say something like, *"Great job! High five!"*—unless that's your inside joke!

Reinvent the Routine

If you feel like you're falling into the same old patterns, find small ways to change things up. A new location, a different time, or even a new playlist can turn something predictable into something unforgettable. Just don't surprise them with a playlist from the 80s unless you both love retro hits!

The Importance of Romance Beyond Sex

Seduce Outside the Bedroom

Being a good lover starts not in bed, but in how you treat your partner day-to-day. Surprise them with something unexpected: coffee at their favorite spot or a hidden note that says, *"I'll see you tonight."* Just don't hide the notes where they might mistake

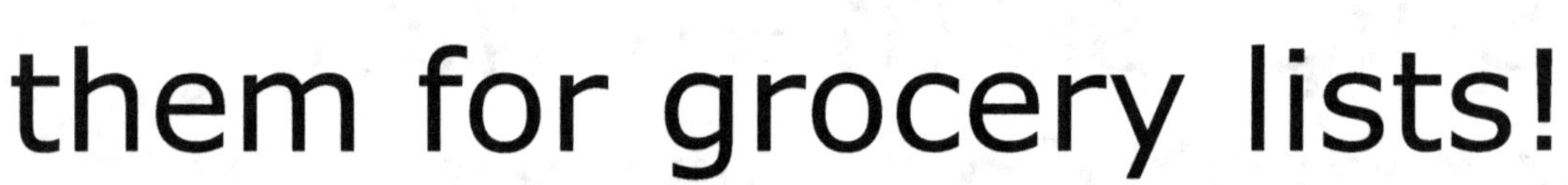

them for grocery lists!

Create a Distraction-Free Environment

Turn off your phone, forget about work, and give them your full attention. Trust me, no *"ping"* from WhatsApp should interrupt something as important as connecting with your partner. Unless it's a message from them— then maybe answer!

Understand That Everyone Is Different

What worked with someone else might not work with your partner. Learn to adapt and personalize the experience. It's like cooking: not all recipes use the same ingredients, and sometimes you need to tweak things to taste!

Never Take Your Partner for Granted

Appreciate the moments you share and make them feel special. A simple *"I love being with you"* can be as powerful as any elaborate technique. Plus, it's easier to say than trying to master a new move!

Vulnerability Is Also Sexy

Showing your emotions, talking about what you feel, or even admitting your nerves can bring you closer to your partner. Emotional connection always amplifies the physical one. Just don't start crying during a romantic movie reenactment!

Emotional and Mental Connection

Listen More Than You Speak

A good lover knows how to listen, not just during pre-sex conversations but also during the act. Your partner's sighs, moans, or even their silence can tell you more than words ever could. Have you ever really listened to the rhythm of their breathing? It might be

more enlightening than
any soundtrack!

Open Mind for New Experiences

New experiences can be intimidating, but they're often what make a relationship unforgettable. Don't be afraid to try something different, whether it's a new position, a different location, or even a type of erotic play you hadn't considered before. Just make sure you're both comfortable—no one wants to end up in an unexpected yoga pose!

Don't Take Everything Too Seriously

Sex should be fun. If something doesn't go as planned, laugh it off, relax, and move forward. Imagine you're an action star in a comedy film instead of a dramatic protagonist. The key is to enjoy, even the awkward moments!

The Power of Small Details

Sometimes, what people remember most isn't what you did, but how you did it. It could be a look, a subtle touch, or a word that leaves a mark. Don't just focus on the action; pay attention to those invisible details that truly make a difference. Just don't try to memorize their favorite color mid-action!

Remember That Desire is Built

Desire doesn't always appear out of nowhere. It's often cultivated throughout the day with small gestures, knowing looks, or playful banter. If you want to increase sexual tension, it's not just about the act itself but creating a buildup filled with expectations.

Make your partner
crave you before even
reaching the bedroom!

The Importance of Patience

Do It at Their Pace

Not all bodies respond the same way or at the same pace. Be patient and listen. Your partner might need more time to reach climax, and that's okay. Patience not only shows you care but also makes the experience much more satisfying for both of you. Think of it as marinating meat—

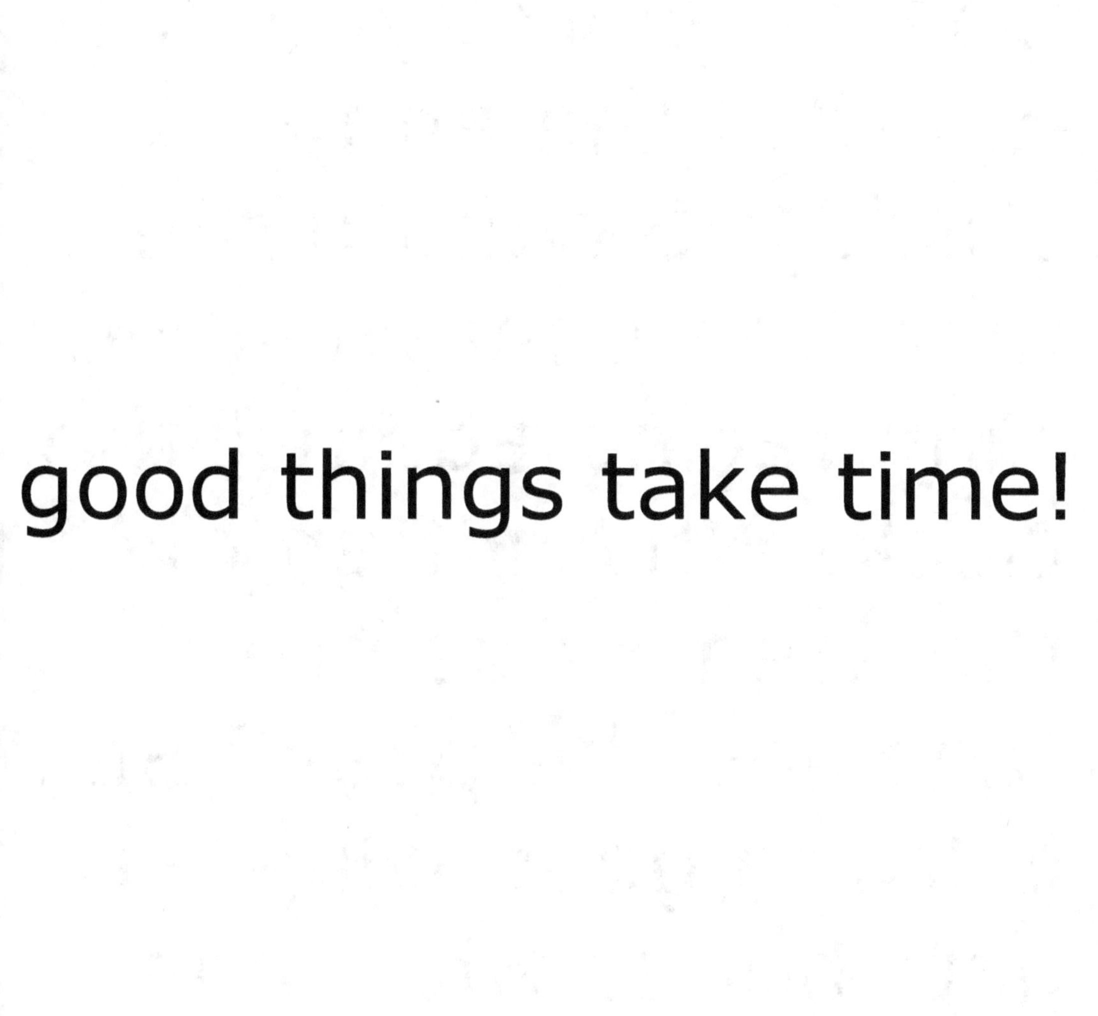

good things take time!

Don't Rush the Finish Line

Don't feel like you need to reach the end quickly. Savoring the moment is much sexier than racing against the clock. Why not enjoy the scenery before reaching the peak? Sex is like a good wine—it gets better with time. Just don't try to pair it with instant noodles!

Respond to Changes in Their Body

Bodies communicate, and a good lover knows how to read that language. If you notice your partner changing their rhythm or posture, they're probably seeking more pleasure. Make sure to adapt to those changes and respond instinctively, without hesitation. It's like dancing—just follow the lead and enjoy the rhythm!

The Importance of Rest

Not everything has to be continuous action. Sometimes, a strategic pause is the best move to recharge and maintain desire for longer. Let the moment become more intense after a brief break. It's like the suspense before a big plot twist in a movie—keeps things exciting!

Fun and Variety in Bed

Sex Isn't a Fixed Formula

There's no *"perfect recipe"* for sex. The right formula is what works for you and your partner in that moment. What worked yesterday might not be needed today. Don't be afraid to mix things up, always respectfully. Just don't try cooking during your

rendezvous!

Try Different Locations

The bed is great, but why not explore new settings? Think the sofa, the shower, or even the kitchen. Sometimes, a simple change of environment can add a spark of excitement. Just make sure there are no dangerous objects nearby... the last time I tried something in the kitchen, I almost broke a glass!

Lingerie, Yes, But with a Surprise

Sexy attire is great, but surprises are even better. You don't need to spend a fortune on underwear. In fact, the best look is an unexpected one: that old t-shirt of your partner that makes them look ten times more attractive. Surprise and cheekiness are the winning combo!

Play with the Senses
Use things that can stimulate other senses like touch and smell. Blindfolds, aromatic oils, or even a bit of melted chocolate can add a whole new level of excitement. Just make sure it doesn't turn into a mess... melted chocolate can be a great ally, but also a great stain!

Self-Care and Well-Being

Take Time for Yourself

Sex is also about how you feel about yourself. Make sure to take care of yourself both physically and mentally. Self-awareness is key, and if you feel good about yourself, you'll transmit that positive energy. And don't forget, a bit of exercise not only improves your health but also your performance in bed. Your body will thank you!

Don't Forget Mental Hygiene

If you have problems or worries that distract you, communicate them. Sometimes, the best thing you can do is let go of what's on your mind to fully enjoy the moment. Mental health is just as important as physical health for a fulfilling experience. Unless you're worried about where you left your keys—then maybe take a quick break to find them!

Learn to Be Flexible

And not just physically. Mental and emotional flexibility is crucial. While your body can adapt to different positions, your mind should also be ready to explore and try new things without judgment or insecurities. It's like stretching before a workout—keeps

everything running
smoothly!

Enjoy Without Pressure

Sometimes we put too much pressure on ourselves to *"do it right"*. Forget about being perfect. Sex should be a pleasurable experience for everyone involved. Relax, be yourself, and enjoy without any pressure. After all, even the best plans can

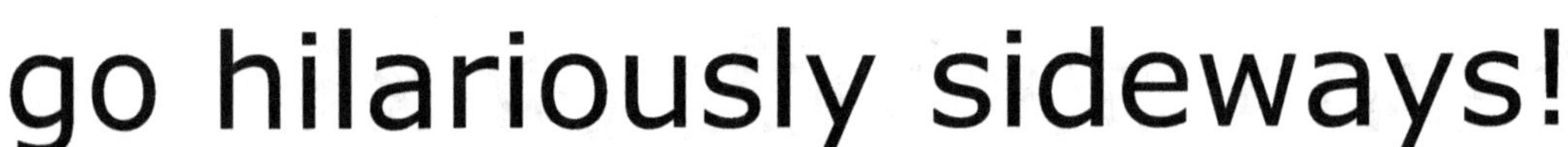

go hilariously sideways!

Ending with the Key to Success

Sex Is a Conversation

It's not all about actions; sometimes words have incredible power. Talking about what you like, what excites you, and how your partner makes you feel creates a deeper connection. Make sure there are always sweet words flowing, both yours and theirs. Just don't turn it into a soap opera!

Curiosity Never Killed the Cat

Always keep your curiosity alive. Ask questions, explore, experiment. The more you discover about what you and your partner enjoy, the more interesting everything becomes. And remember: exploration never ends because there's always something new to learn. Just don't explore underwater unless you both have scuba gear!

Whisper Like a Secret Agent

Use your voice wisely. A soft whisper in their ear can be electrifying. But don't overdo it and start narrating like a spy on a mission—keep it sensual, not suspicious.

Create Your Secret Code

Establish a unique gesture or phrase that only the two of you understand. Whether it's a wink or "the laundry needs folding," it'll be your discreet way of saying, "Let's make magic tonight."

Take the Compliment Game Further

Compliments are great, but go beyond the usual "you're amazing." Try specifics like, "The way you smiled during that moment... unforgettable!" But don't overdo it, or they'll think you're writing a Yelp review.